Pollen Power Harnessing the Benefits of Bee Pollen

By

Alex Lenero

I am pleased to present my latest book to you, in which I have poured my heart and soul. I hope it has captured your imagination and provided you with valuable insights and entertainment. My writing style for guides is simple and straightforward, removing all the excess that many books tend to have.

If you enjoyed this book, I invite you to explore my other works. I have written on various topics, both fiction and non-fiction, and I believe there is something in my catalog for every reader. You can find all my books on Amazon Kindle.

In addition to my books, I also have a blog at theuniversaloracle.com where I share my reflections and thoughts on various topics. Whether you are looking for inspiration, information, or simply a good read, I am confident that you will find something interesting on my blog

I sincerely appreciate you taking the time to read this book and consider my other works. Your support means a lot to me and I hope to hear from you soon.

Best regards,

Alex Lenero

Contents

Introduction

Welcome to "Pollen Power: Harnessing the Benefits of Bee Pollen". In this book, we will explore the health benefits of bee pollen and its potential to support overall health and wellness. Bee pollen has been used as a natural supplement for centuries, and recent research has begun to shed light on its many potential health benefits.

Bee pollen is a natural substance produced by bees as they collect nectar from flowers. It is a rich source of nutrients, including protein, vitamins, minerals, and antioxidants. Many people believe that bee pollen can be used to support the immune system, promote healthy digestion, and improve energy levels.

This book is designed to provide a comprehensive overview of the potential health benefits of bee pollen. We will explore the scientific evidence on its effects, drawing on insights from nutrition, biochemistry, and related disciplines. We will also provide practical tips for incorporating bee pollen into your diet, as well as guidance on choosing high-quality bee pollen supplements.

What is Bee Pollen?

Bee pollen is a natural substance produced by bees as they collect nectar from flowers. It is a powdery substance made up of pollen grains, nectar, enzymes, and wax. Bees collect the pollen on their bodies as they move from flower to flower, and then pack it into small pellets to take back to the hive.

Bee pollen is a rich source of nutrients, including protein, vitamins, minerals, and antioxidants. It has been used as a natural supplement for centuries, with many people believing that it can help to support overall health and wellness.

The composition of bee pollen can vary depending on the types of plants and flowers that the bees are collecting from. However, bee pollen typically contains a wide range of nutrients, including essential amino acids, fatty acids, vitamins (such as vitamin C and vitamin E), minerals (such as calcium, iron, and zinc), and antioxidants (such as flavonoids and carotenoids).

In recent years, researchers have begun to explore the potential health benefits of bee pollen. While the scientific evidence is still emerging, some studies have suggested that bee pollen may have a range of health-promoting effects, including supporting the immune system, promoting healthy digestion, and improving energy levels.

Overall, bee pollen is a fascinating and promising natural substance that has the potential to support overall health and wellness. In the following chapters of "Pollen Power: Harnessing the Benefits of Bee Pollen", we will explore the science behind bee pollen and the many potential health benefits it may offer.

The Nutritional Value of Bee Pollen

Bee pollen is a nutrient-dense food that is rich in a wide range of essential vitamins, minerals, and other nutrients. It is considered to be one of the most nutritionally complete natural substances in the world. The exact nutritional composition of bee pollen can vary depending on the types of plants and flowers that the bees are collecting from, but it typically contains a range of nutrients, including:

1. Protein: Bee pollen is a rich source of protein, which is essential for building and repairing tissues in the body. It contains all 22 amino acids, including 8 essential amino acids that the body cannot produce on its own.

2. Vitamins: Bee pollen contains a wide range of vitamins, including vitamins A, C, D, E, and K, as well as the B vitamins. These vitamins play a critical role in many bodily processes, including supporting immune function, promoting healthy skin and eyesight, and aiding in the metabolism of nutrients.

3. Minerals: Bee pollen is also a good source of minerals, including calcium, magnesium, potassium, and zinc. These minerals are essential for maintaining healthy bones, muscles, and other bodily functions.

4. Enzymes: Bee pollen contains a range of enzymes that are important for digestion and nutrient absorption. These enzymes can help to break

down food more efficiently and make nutrients more bioavailable to the body.

5. Antioxidants: Bee pollen is rich in antioxidants, which can help to protect the body against oxidative stress and damage caused by free radicals. These antioxidants include flavonoids, carotenoids, and other compounds that have been shown to have anti-inflammatory and anti-cancer properties.

Overall, bee pollen is a highly nutritious food that offers a wide range of health benefits. In the following chapters of "Pollen Power: Harnessing the Benefits of Bee Pollen", we will explore the specific nutritional benefits of bee pollen in more detail, as well as the potential health effects it may offer.

The Health Benefits of Bee Pollen

Bee pollen has been traditionally used as a natural supplement to support overall health and wellness. While the scientific evidence on the health benefits of bee pollen is still emerging, some studies have suggested that bee pollen may offer a range of health-promoting effects. Here are some potential health benefits of bee pollen:

1. Immune system support: Bee pollen is rich in antioxidants and other compounds that have been shown to support the immune system. It may help to reduce inflammation and protect the body against oxidative stress, which can lead to chronic diseases.

2. Digestive health: Bee pollen may also help to promote healthy digestion. It contains enzymes and other compounds that can help to break down food and improve nutrient absorption. Some studies have suggested that bee pollen may also have anti-inflammatory effects on the digestive system.

3. Energy and vitality: Bee pollen is a natural source of energy, and may help to improve stamina and reduce fatigue. It contains a range of nutrients, including vitamins and minerals, that can help to support overall energy levels.

4. Skin and hair health: Bee pollen may also have benefits for the skin and hair. It contains compounds that have been shown to have anti-inflammatory and antioxidant properties, which

can help to protect the skin against damage and support healthy hair growth.

5. Other health benefits: Bee pollen has been traditionally used for a wide range of health conditions, including allergies, asthma, and liver disease. While the scientific evidence on these uses is still limited, some studies have suggested that bee pollen may have potential benefits for these conditions.

Overall, bee pollen is a promising natural substance that has the potential to offer a range of health benefits. In the following chapters of "Pollen Power: Harnessing the Benefits of Bee Pollen", we will explore the specific health benefits of bee pollen in more detail, drawing on the latest research and scholarship in this field.

The Science of Bee Pollen

The science of bee pollen is a fascinating and rapidly evolving area of study, as researchers seek to understand the composition and potential health benefits of this natural substance. Here are some key insights into the science of bee pollen:

1. The composition of bee pollen: Bee pollen is a complex substance made up of pollen grains, nectar, enzymes, and wax. The exact composition of bee pollen can vary depending on the types of plants and flowers that the bees are collecting from. However, bee pollen typically contains a wide range of nutrients, including essential amino acids, fatty acids, vitamins (such as vitamin C and vitamin E), minerals (such as calcium, iron, and zinc), and antioxidants (such as flavonoids and carotenoids).

2. How bee pollen is collected and processed: Bees collect pollen on their bodies as they move from flower to flower, and then pack it into small pellets to take back to the hive. Once back at the hive, the pollen is mixed with nectar and enzymes and packed into cells in the honeycomb. Over time, the mixture is dried and becomes a solid substance that can be harvested and used.

3. The role of bee pollen in the environment: Bee pollen plays a critical role in the environment, as it is a key source of nutrients for bees and other insects. It also plays a role in plant reproduction, as bees collect pollen from one flower and transfer it to another, allowing for pollination to occur.

4. Potential health benefits: While the scientific evidence on the health benefits of bee pollen is

still emerging, some studies have suggested that bee pollen may have a range of health-promoting effects, including supporting the immune system, promoting healthy digestion, and improving energy levels.

Overall, the science of bee pollen is a complex and rapidly evolving field, as researchers seek to understand the composition and potential health benefits of this fascinating natural substance. In the following chapters of "Pollen Power: Harnessing the Benefits of Bee Pollen", we will explore the science behind bee pollen in more detail, drawing on insights from nutrition, biochemistry, and related fields to develop a comprehensive understanding of this natural substance.

How Bee Pollen is Collected and Processed

Bee pollen is collected by worker bees as they fly from flower to flower in search of nectar. As they collect nectar, the bees also collect pollen grains on their bodies, which they pack into small pellets using their legs and mouthparts. The bees then carry the pollen pellets back to the hive, where they are stored in honeycomb cells.

Once back at the hive, the bee pollen is mixed with nectar, enzymes, and bee saliva to create a mixture that is more easily digestible. The mixture is then packed into the cells of the honeycomb, where it is left to dry and ferment. This process can take several days, during which time the bee pollen becomes more concentrated and more nutritious.

To collect bee pollen for human consumption, beekeepers use specially designed traps that are placed at the entrance of the hive. These traps allow the bees to enter and exit the hive freely, but collect the pollen pellets as they do so. The collected pollen is then processed to remove any debris or impurities, and may be dried or frozen to preserve its nutritional content.

It's important to note that not all bee pollen is created equal, and the quality of bee pollen can vary depending on a number of factors, including the types of plants and flowers that the bees are collecting from, the harvesting and processing methods used, and the storage conditions. To ensure that you are getting high-quality bee pollen, it's important to choose a reputable source and to look for products that have been tested for purity and quality.

The Role of Bee Pollen in the Environment

Bee pollen plays a critical role in the environment, as it is a key source of nutrients for bees and other insects. Bees collect pollen from flowers as they move from plant to plant in search of nectar. As they collect pollen, they inadvertently transfer pollen from one flower to another, allowing for cross-pollination to occur. This process is essential for the reproduction of many plant species, including many of the fruits and vegetables that we rely on for food.

In addition to supporting plant reproduction, bee pollen also plays a key role in the ecosystem by providing a rich source of nutrition for bees and other insects. Bees use pollen as a source of protein and other essential nutrients to support their growth and reproduction. In fact, bee pollen is often referred to as "bee bread" because it is so essential to the survival of the hive.

Beyond bees, many other species of insects also rely on pollen as a source of nutrition. Pollen is a rich source of protein, vitamins, and minerals, and provides essential nutrients for many insects, including butterflies, moths, and beetles.

Overall, the role of bee pollen in the environment is essential for supporting the health and survival of many plant and animal species. By providing a rich source of nutrition and supporting cross-pollination, bee pollen plays a critical role in maintaining the health and diversity of ecosystems around the world.

Incorporating Bee Pollen into Your Diet

Incorporating bee pollen into your diet is a great way to take advantage of its many nutritional benefits. Here are some tips for incorporating bee pollen into your diet:

1. Start with a small amount: If you are new to bee pollen, start with a small amount to see how your body reacts. A good starting point is 1/4 to 1/2 teaspoon per day.

2. Use bee pollen as a topping: Bee pollen has a sweet and slightly floral taste that makes it a great topping for yogurt, smoothie bowls, oatmeal, or other breakfast foods.

3. Mix it into a salad dressing: Bee pollen can also be mixed into a salad dressing for an extra boost of nutrition. Simply mix it with olive oil, vinegar, and your favorite herbs and spices.

4. Add it to baked goods: Bee pollen can also be added to baked goods like muffins or granola bars. It adds a nice crunch and a boost of nutrition to your favorite recipes.

5. Use it as a natural sweetener: Bee pollen can be used as a natural sweetener in recipes like smoothies or tea. It has a slightly sweet taste that can help to reduce the need for added sugars.

6. Choose high-quality sources: When purchasing bee pollen, look for high-quality sources that have been tested for purity and quality. Be sure to choose a reputable brand that follows good

manufacturing practices to ensure that you are getting a safe and high-quality product.

Overall, incorporating bee pollen into your diet is a great way to take advantage of its many nutritional benefits. It's a versatile ingredient that can be used in a variety of ways to add nutrition and flavor to your favorite foods.

Choosing High-Quality Bee Pollen

Choosing high-quality bee pollen is essential to ensure that you are getting a safe and nutritious product. Here are some tips for choosing high-quality bee pollen:

1. Look for organic sources: Choose bee pollen that comes from organic sources, which are free from pesticides and other harmful chemicals. This ensures that you are getting a pure and natural product.

2. Choose reputable brands: Choose bee pollen from reputable brands that follow good manufacturing practices. Look for companies that have a strong track record of producing high-quality, safe, and effective products.

3. Check for purity: Look for bee pollen that has been tested for purity, which ensures that it is free from contaminants and other impurities. Many reputable brands will provide information on their testing procedures and the results of their tests.

4. Consider the source: Consider where the bee pollen comes from. Bee pollen that comes from diverse sources is likely to have a wider range of nutrients and other beneficial compounds.

5. Check the color and texture: High-quality bee pollen should have a vibrant color and a slightly sweet, floral aroma. It should have a fine, powdery texture and should not be clumpy or sticky.

6. Check the expiration date: Bee pollen is a natural product and can spoil over time. Make sure to check the expiration date before purchasing, and only buy bee pollen that is fresh and within its expiration date.

By following these tips, you can ensure that you are getting a high-quality, safe, and nutritious product when purchasing bee pollen.

How to Use Bee Pollen

Bee pollen can be used in a variety of ways to add nutrition and flavor to your favorite foods. Here are some ways to use bee pollen:

1. As a topping: Bee pollen has a sweet, slightly floral taste that makes it a great topping for yogurt, smoothie bowls, oatmeal, or other breakfast foods.

2. In smoothies: Bee pollen can be blended into smoothies for an extra boost of nutrition. It can also add a nice texture and flavor to your favorite smoothie recipes.

3. In salad dressings: Bee pollen can be mixed into a salad dressing for an extra boost of nutrition. Simply mix it with olive oil, vinegar, and your favorite herbs and spices.

4. In baked goods: Bee pollen can be added to baked goods like muffins or granola bars. It adds a nice crunch and a boost of nutrition to your favorite recipes.

5. As a natural sweetener: Bee pollen can be used as a natural sweetener in recipes like smoothies or tea. It has a slightly sweet taste that can help to reduce the need for added sugars.

6. Sprinkled on fruit: Bee pollen can be sprinkled on top of fresh fruit for a tasty and nutritious snack.

7. In tea: Bee pollen can be added to hot or cold tea for an extra boost of nutrition. Simply stir in a small amount of bee pollen until it dissolves.

When using bee pollen, it's important to start with a small amount to see how your body reacts. If you have any allergies to bee products or pollen, it's important to speak with your healthcare provider before using bee pollen. Additionally, be sure to choose a high-quality, pure product to ensure that you are getting the full range of benefits from bee pollen.

Recipes for Incorporating Bee Pollen into Your Diet

Here are some recipes for incorporating bee pollen into your diet:

1. Bee Pollen Yogurt Bowl:

- 1 cup Greek yogurt

- 1 banana, sliced

- 1/4 cup blueberries

- 1 tablespoon bee pollen

Instructions:

1. Add the Greek yogurt to a bowl.

2. Top with sliced banana, blueberries, and bee pollen.

3. Serve and enjoy!

4. Bee Pollen Smoothie:

- 1 banana

- 1/2 cup frozen berries

- 1/2 cup almond milk

- 1 tablespoon bee pollen

Instructions:

1. Add all ingredients to a blender and blend until smooth.

2. Pour into a glass and enjoy!

3. Bee Pollen Salad Dressing:

- 1/4 cup olive oil

- 2 tablespoons apple cider vinegar

- 1 teaspoon honey

- 1 teaspoon Dijon mustard

- 1 teaspoon bee pollen

- Salt and pepper to taste

Instructions:

1. In a small bowl, whisk together the olive oil, apple cider vinegar, honey, and Dijon mustard.

2. Add the bee pollen and whisk to combine.

3. Season with salt and pepper to taste.

4. Drizzle the dressing over your favorite salad and enjoy!

5. Bee Pollen Energy Balls:

- 1 cup pitted dates

- 1/2 cup almonds

- 1/4 cup rolled oats

- 2 tablespoons chia seeds

- 2 tablespoons bee pollen

- 1/2 teaspoon vanilla extract

- Pinch of salt

Instructions:

1. Add all ingredients to a food processor and pulse until the mixture is finely chopped and sticks together.

2. Roll the mixture into balls and refrigerate until firm.

3. Serve and enjoy!

These are just a few examples of recipes for incorporating bee pollen into your diet. Bee pollen is a versatile ingredient that can be used in a variety of ways to add nutrition and flavor to your favorite foods. Experiment with different recipes and find what works best for you!

Immune System Support

Bee pollen has been shown to have a number of potential benefits for immune system support. Here are some of the ways that bee pollen may help support immune function:

1. Antioxidant properties: Bee pollen contains a range of antioxidants, including flavonoids and carotenoids. These antioxidants can help to protect the body against oxidative stress and damage caused by free radicals. This can help to support immune function by reducing inflammation and preventing damage to cells and tissues.

2. Anti-inflammatory properties: Bee pollen has been shown to have anti-inflammatory properties, which can help to reduce inflammation in the body. This is important for supporting immune function, as chronic inflammation can impair the body's ability to fight off infections and other threats.

3. Immunomodulatory effects: Bee pollen has been shown to have immunomodulatory effects, meaning that it can help to regulate immune function. It has been shown to stimulate the production of immune cells and antibodies, which can help to boost the body's natural defenses against infection.

4. Nutritional support: Bee pollen is a rich source of nutrients, including vitamins, minerals, and amino acids. These nutrients are essential for supporting immune function, as they help to provide the building blocks needed for the production of immune cells and other components of the immune system.

Overall, bee pollen may help to support immune function by providing a range of beneficial compounds that can reduce inflammation, protect against oxidative stress, and stimulate the production of immune cells and antibodies. However, more research is needed to fully understand the potential benefits of bee pollen for immune system support. If you have any questions or concerns about using bee pollen for immune support, it's important to speak with your healthcare provider.

Digestive Health

Bee pollen has been shown to have potential benefits for digestive health. Here are some of the ways that bee pollen may help support digestive function:

1. Probiotic properties: Bee pollen has been shown to have probiotic properties, meaning that it can help to support the growth of beneficial bacteria in the gut. This can help to promote digestive health by improving the balance of gut bacteria and supporting healthy digestion.

2. Anti-inflammatory properties: Bee pollen has been shown to have anti-inflammatory properties, which can help to reduce inflammation in the gut. This is important for supporting digestive health, as chronic inflammation in the gut can lead to a range of digestive issues.

3. Nutritional support: Bee pollen is a rich source of nutrients, including vitamins, minerals, and amino acids. These nutrients are essential for supporting digestive function, as they help to provide the building blocks needed for the production of digestive enzymes and other components of the digestive system.

4. Digestive enzyme support: Bee pollen has been shown to contain a range of digestive enzymes, including amylase, lipase, and protease. These enzymes can help to support healthy digestion by breaking down carbohydrates, fats, and proteins into smaller, more easily digestible molecules.

Overall, bee pollen may help to support digestive function by providing probiotic and anti-inflammatory properties, as well as a range of beneficial nutrients and digestive enzymes. However, more research is needed to fully understand the potential benefits of bee pollen for digestive health. If you have any questions or concerns about using bee pollen for digestive support, it's important to speak with your healthcare provider.

Energy and Vitality

Bee pollen has been shown to have potential benefits for energy and vitality. Here are some of the ways that bee pollen may help support energy and vitality:

1. Nutritional support: Bee pollen is a rich source of nutrients, including vitamins, minerals, and amino acids. These nutrients are essential for supporting energy production, as they help to provide the building blocks needed for the production of ATP (the body's main source of energy).

2. Adaptogenic properties: Bee pollen has been shown to have adaptogenic properties, meaning that it can help the body to adapt to stress and support healthy energy levels. Adaptogens can help to balance hormones and reduce fatigue, which can help to support energy and vitality.

3. Anti-inflammatory properties: Bee pollen has been shown to have anti-inflammatory properties, which can help to reduce inflammation in the body. This is important for supporting energy and vitality, as chronic inflammation can lead to fatigue and other symptoms.

4. Antioxidant properties: Bee pollen contains a range of antioxidants, including flavonoids and carotenoids. These antioxidants can help to protect the body against oxidative stress and damage caused by free radicals. This can help to support energy and vitality by reducing inflammation and preventing damage to cells and tissues.

Overall, bee pollen may help to support energy and vitality by providing a range of beneficial compounds that can support healthy energy levels and reduce fatigue. However, more research is needed to fully understand the potential benefits of bee pollen for energy and vitality. If you have any questions or concerns about using bee pollen for energy support, it's important to speak with your healthcare provider.

Skin and Hair Health

Bee pollen has been shown to have potential benefits for skin and hair health. Here are some of the ways that bee pollen may help support healthy skin and hair:

1. Anti-inflammatory properties: Bee pollen has been shown to have anti-inflammatory properties, which can help to reduce inflammation in the skin. This is important for supporting healthy skin and hair, as chronic inflammation can lead to a range of skin and hair issues.

2. Antioxidant properties: Bee pollen contains a range of antioxidants, including flavonoids and carotenoids. These antioxidants can help to protect the skin and hair against oxidative stress and damage caused by free radicals.

3. Nutritional support: Bee pollen is a rich source of nutrients, including vitamins, minerals, and amino acids. These nutrients are essential for supporting healthy skin and hair, as they help to provide the building blocks needed for the production of collagen, keratin, and other components of the skin and hair.

4. Moisturizing properties: Bee pollen has been shown to have moisturizing properties, which can help to hydrate and nourish the skin and hair.

5. Antibacterial properties: Bee pollen has been shown to have antibacterial properties, which can help to protect the skin and hair against bacterial infections and other issues.

Overall, bee pollen may help to support healthy skin and hair by providing anti-inflammatory, antioxidant, nutritional, moisturizing, and antibacterial properties. However, more research is needed to fully understand the potential benefits of bee pollen for skin and hair health. If you have any questions or concerns about using bee pollen for skin or hair support, it's important to speak with your healthcare provider.

Other Health Benefits of Bee Pollen

In addition to the benefits mentioned earlier, bee pollen has been studied for its potential benefits on a variety of other health conditions, such as:

1. Allergies: Some studies suggest that bee pollen may help to reduce the symptoms of allergies, such as hay fever, by helping the body to build up a tolerance to allergens.

2. Cardiovascular health: Bee pollen has been shown to have potential benefits for cardiovascular health, including reducing inflammation and oxidative stress, and improving blood lipid profiles.

3. Athletic performance: Bee pollen has been shown to have potential benefits for athletic performance, including reducing muscle fatigue and improving endurance.

4. Menopausal symptoms: Bee pollen has been studied for its potential benefits on menopausal symptoms, such as hot flashes and mood changes.

5. Cancer: Some studies have suggested that bee pollen may have potential anti-cancer properties, although more research is needed in this area.

It's important to note that many of these potential benefits are based on preliminary research, and more studies are needed to fully understand the effects of bee pollen on these health conditions. If you have any questions or concerns about using bee pollen for a specific health condition, it's important to speak with your healthcare provider.

Bee Pollen Supplements

Bee pollen supplements are available in a variety of forms, including capsules, tablets, and powders. These supplements are typically made from dried and ground bee pollen, and may be combined with other ingredients or sold as a standalone product.

When choosing a bee pollen supplement, it's important to choose a high-quality product that has been tested for purity and potency. Look for products that have been certified by a third-party testing organization, and that provide information on the source of the bee pollen, the processing methods used, and the nutritional content of the supplement.

It's also important to be aware of any potential side effects or allergic reactions associated with bee pollen supplements. Some people may be allergic to bee pollen, and may experience symptoms such as hives, swelling, or difficulty breathing when using bee pollen supplements. Additionally, bee pollen may interact with certain medications, so it's important to speak with your healthcare provider before using bee pollen supplements if you are taking any prescription or over-the-counter medications.

Overall, bee pollen supplements can be a convenient way to incorporate bee pollen into your diet and support your health. However, it's important to choose a high-quality product and to be aware of any potential side effects or interactions with medications.

Types of Bee Pollen Supplements

Bee pollen supplements are available in a variety of forms, including:

1. Capsules: Bee pollen capsules contain dried and ground bee pollen, typically in a gelatin or vegetarian capsule.

2. Tablets: Bee pollen tablets are similar to capsules, but are pressed into a solid tablet form instead.

3. Powder: Bee pollen powder is made from ground bee pollen and can be added to smoothies, yogurt, or other foods.

4. Granules: Bee pollen granules are small, hard pellets of bee pollen that can be sprinkled on top of food or eaten on their own.

5. Liquid extract: Some bee pollen supplements come in liquid extract form, which can be added to water or other beverages.

When choosing a bee pollen supplement, it's important to consider factors such as purity, potency, and sourcing. Look for products that have been certified by a third-party testing organization, and that provide information on the source of the bee pollen, the processing methods used, and the nutritional content of the supplement. Additionally, be aware of any potential side effects or interactions with medications, and speak with your healthcare provider before using bee pollen supplements if you have any concerns or questions.

Choosing the Right Bee Pollen Supplement

Choosing the right bee pollen supplement can be challenging, as there are many different products available on the market. Here are some factors to consider when choosing a bee pollen supplement:

1. Quality and Purity: Look for a supplement that has been tested for purity and quality. The supplement should be free of contaminants, such as heavy metals, pesticides, and other toxins.

2. Sourcing: The source of the bee pollen is important. Choose a product that comes from a reputable source and is sustainably harvested.

3. Processing Method: The processing method used to create the supplement can affect the quality of the product. Look for a supplement that uses a gentle processing method, such as freeze-drying, which helps to preserve the nutrients in the bee pollen.

4. Nutritional Content: Look for a supplement that provides detailed information about the nutritional content of the bee pollen, including the levels of vitamins, minerals, and amino acids.

5. Form: Consider the form of the supplement that will be most convenient for you. Capsules and tablets may be easier to take on-the-go, while powders and granules may be more versatile for adding to recipes.

6. Allergies: If you have a history of allergies, particularly to bee products, it's important to speak

with your healthcare provider before using a bee
pollen supplement.

Ultimately, choosing the right bee pollen supplement
requires careful consideration of the factors above. Be
sure to do your research and choose a high-quality
product from a reputable source to ensure you are getting
the maximum benefits from bee pollen.

How to Take Bee Pollen Supplements

The method for taking bee pollen supplements may depend on the type of supplement you choose. Here are some general guidelines for taking bee pollen supplements:

1. Capsules and Tablets: Follow the manufacturer's instructions for the recommended dosage. Typically, this will involve taking one to three capsules or tablets per day, with or without food.

2. Powder: Bee pollen powder can be added to smoothies, yogurt, oatmeal, or other foods. Start with a small amount and gradually increase the dosage as needed.

3. Granules: Bee pollen granules can be added to salads, cereal, or other foods. Start with a small amount and gradually increase the dosage as needed.

4. Liquid Extract: Follow the manufacturer's instructions for the recommended dosage. Typically, this will involve adding a few drops of liquid extract to water or another beverage.

It's important to start with a small dosage of bee pollen supplements and gradually increase the dosage as needed. This will help to minimize the risk of allergic reactions or other side effects. It's also important to speak with your healthcare provider before taking bee pollen supplements, especially if you are taking any prescription or over-the-counter medications, or if you have a history of allergies. Finally, be sure to choose a high-quality product from a reputable source to ensure you are getting the maximum benefits from bee pollen.

Precautions and Considerations

While bee pollen supplements can be a convenient way to incorporate bee pollen into your diet and support your health, there are some precautions and considerations to keep in mind:

1. Allergies: Some people may be allergic to bee pollen, and may experience symptoms such as hives, swelling, or difficulty breathing when using bee pollen supplements. If you have a history of allergies, especially to bee products, it's important to speak with your healthcare provider before using bee pollen supplements.

2. Interactions with Medications: Bee pollen may interact with certain medications, such as blood thinners, and may affect the absorption and metabolism of other medications. If you are taking any prescription or over-the-counter medications, it's important to speak with your healthcare provider before using bee pollen supplements.

3. Quality and Purity: The quality and purity of bee pollen supplements can vary widely. Look for products that have been tested for purity and quality, and that provide detailed information on the source and processing of the bee pollen.

4. Dosage: It's important to start with a small dosage of bee pollen supplements and gradually increase the dosage as needed. This will help to minimize the risk of allergic reactions or other side effects.

5. Children and Pregnant Women: Bee pollen
    supplements are not recommended for children or
    pregnant women, as the potential risks and
    benefits are not well understood.

Overall, while bee pollen supplements can be a beneficial
addition to a healthy diet, it's important to be aware of the
potential risks and to speak with your healthcare provider
before using bee pollen supplements. By following these
precautions and considerations, you can make an
informed decision about whether bee pollen supplements
are right for you.

Possible Allergic Reaction

Bee pollen can cause allergic reactions in some people, particularly those who are allergic to bee products. Symptoms of an allergic reaction to bee pollen can include:

1. Hives or skin rash

2. Itching or swelling, especially around the mouth or throat

3. Difficulty breathing or tightness in the chest

4. Dizziness or lightheadedness

5. Nausea or vomiting

If you experience any of these symptoms after taking a bee pollen supplement, it's important to stop taking the supplement and seek medical attention immediately. In severe cases, an allergic reaction to bee pollen can be life-threatening and may require emergency medical treatment.

It's also important to note that even if you don't have a known allergy to bee products, it's still possible to develop an allergy to bee pollen. If you are using bee pollen supplements for the first time, it's important to start with a small dosage and monitor your body's response. If you experience any symptoms of an allergic reaction, stop taking the supplement and speak with your healthcare provider.

In general, bee pollen supplements should be used with caution by people with a history of allergies, and it's important to speak with your healthcare provider before using bee pollen supplements if you have any concerns or questions.

Interactions with Medications

Bee pollen may interact with certain medications, including:

1. Blood Thinners: Bee pollen may have anticoagulant properties, which can increase the risk of bleeding in people taking blood thinners, such as warfarin or aspirin.

2. Immunosuppressants: Bee pollen may stimulate the immune system, which can interfere with the effectiveness of immunosuppressive medications, such as cyclosporine or tacrolimus.

3. Hormones: Bee pollen may have estrogen-like effects, which can interfere with the effectiveness of hormone medications, such as birth control pills or hormone replacement therapy.

4. Antibiotics: Bee pollen may interfere with the absorption and effectiveness of antibiotics, such as tetracycline or penicillin.

If you are taking any prescription or over-the-counter medications, it's important to speak with your healthcare provider before using bee pollen supplements. They can advise you on any potential interactions and help you determine whether bee pollen supplements are safe for you to use.

In general, it's important to be cautious when combining supplements and medications, as interactions can occur and may have serious health consequences. If you have any concerns or questions about the safety of using bee pollen supplements with your current medications, speak with your healthcare provider before starting a new supplement regimen.

Pregnancy and Nursing

Bee pollen supplements are not recommended for pregnant or nursing women, as the potential risks and benefits are not well understood. While bee pollen is a natural and nutrient-rich food, it's important to be cautious when using supplements during pregnancy and breastfeeding.

Bee pollen may contain contaminants or allergens that could be harmful to a developing fetus or nursing infant. Additionally, bee pollen may stimulate the immune system, which could have potential effects on pregnancy outcomes.

If you are pregnant or nursing, it's important to speak with your healthcare provider before using bee pollen supplements. They can advise you on the potential risks and benefits, and help you determine whether bee pollen supplements are safe for you to use.

In general, it's important to be cautious when using any supplements during pregnancy and breastfeeding. While some supplements may be safe and beneficial, others may have potential risks or side effects. By speaking with your healthcare provider and making informed decisions, you can ensure the health and safety of yourself and your baby.

Conclusion

Bee pollen is a natural and nutrient-rich food that has been used for centuries to support health and wellness. It contains a wide variety of vitamins, minerals, and other nutrients that can help to boost the immune system, support digestive health, and improve energy and vitality.

While bee pollen supplements can be a convenient way to incorporate bee pollen into your diet, it's important to be aware of the potential risks and to choose a high-quality product from a reputable source. Some people may be allergic to bee pollen, and bee pollen may interact with certain medications, so it's important to speak with your healthcare provider before using bee pollen supplements.

In addition, bee pollen supplements are not recommended for pregnant or nursing women, and should be used with caution by people with a history of allergies. By following these precautions and considerations, you can make an informed decision about whether bee pollen supplements are right for you.

Overall, bee pollen is a powerful and natural source of nutrition that can help to support your health and wellness. By incorporating bee pollen into your diet and using supplements with caution, you can reap the many benefits of this powerful superfood.

Recap of Bee Pollen Benefits

Bee pollen is a nutrient-rich superfood that has been used for centuries to support health and wellness. Here is a recap of some of the key benefits of bee pollen:

1. Immune System Support: Bee pollen contains a variety of vitamins, minerals, and other nutrients that can help to boost the immune system and support overall health.

2. Digestive Health: Bee pollen may help to support digestive health by promoting the growth of healthy gut bacteria and reducing inflammation in the digestive tract.

3. Energy and Vitality: Bee pollen can help to boost energy and vitality, thanks to its high nutrient content and ability to support healthy metabolic function.

4. Skin and Hair Health: Bee pollen contains antioxidants and other nutrients that can help to support healthy skin and hair.

5. Other Health Benefits: Bee pollen may have a variety of other health benefits, including reducing inflammation, supporting cardiovascular health, and improving athletic performance.

While bee pollen supplements can be a convenient way to incorporate bee pollen into your diet, it's important to be aware of the potential risks and to choose a high-quality product from a reputable source. If you are considering using bee pollen supplements, speak with your healthcare

provider to determine whether they are safe and
appropriate for you

Final Thoughts and Recommendations

Bee pollen is a natural and nutrient-rich superfood that can provide a variety of health benefits, from immune system support to improved skin and hair health. However, it's important to be aware of the potential risks and to choose a high-quality product from a reputable source.

If you are considering using bee pollen supplements, it's important to speak with your healthcare provider to determine whether they are safe and appropriate for you. You should also be cautious when combining supplements and medications, as interactions can occur and may have serious health consequences.

In addition to bee pollen supplements, you can also incorporate bee pollen into your diet by adding it to smoothies, oatmeal, yogurt, or other foods. Bee pollen is a versatile ingredient that can add a delicious and nutritious boost to a variety of dishes.

Overall, bee pollen can be a powerful and natural way to support your health and wellness. By choosing a high-quality product, using supplements with caution, and incorporating bee pollen into your diet, you can reap the many benefits of this nutrient-rich superfood.